LIVE, LIFE & VEGAN: BECAUSE YOU GIVE A SHIT

Light and Healthy ways to enjoy vegan recipes at any time of the day

By Rose C. Loh

Foreword

This book *"LIVE, LIFE & VEGAN: BECAUSE YOU GIVE A SHIT: Light and Healthy ways to enjoy vegan recipes at any time of the day"* is my gift to you so that you can eat vegetarian food in the most delicious and fuss free manner!

What comes to your mind when you first think about going vegan?

Tasty food? Health? Beauty? Budgeted meals? Or just about anything else!

Many people worry whether they will end up eating boring, bland meals or will run out of ideas and be in a muddle trying to come up with a variety of nutritious vegan recipes that will appeal to each and every member of the family.

True, this can be quite the monumental task. But it is no different from the struggle of "traditional" home chefs around the world.

Finding a variety of delicious vegan meals can be easy, but:

First, we first need to change our mindset and understand why we need to become vegan.

Second, we need to have the willpower to spend a bit more time in the kitchen and prepare wholesome delicious recipes.

Why should you own this cookbook?

- It teaches the truth about being vegan.

- Shows you how you can create balanced meals by simple being Vegan.

- Offers delicious alternatives to certain food items like eggs, meats, and dairy.

- Teaches the long-term benefits of being Vegan both for health reasons and as a responsible individual in this world.

- Lastly, because I have summed up 30 wise steps for hearty recipes for you to jumpstart your path to a nutritious Vegan Life. The recipes consist of Breakfast, Lunch, Dinner, Cravings, Protein Shakes and even Desserts!

Go ahead and make this book a part of your life today and you will understand what I mean. I am on this journey with you!

Table of Contents

Introduction

Being Vegan is sort of the blooming trend nowadays. You have to understand that being Vegan will mean a complete change from your current food patterns. So, it is a change of lifestyle, thoughts, expression, and finally, do trust me, you will be transformed into a cleaner and humbler 'You.'

This book will help you to:

- Understand what sort of vitamins and minerals are contained in each and every vegetable you take and then show you how to reorganize your meal plans and recipes accordingly.

- A list of pure vegetarian alternatives to some ingredients (like eggs) have been included in this book. This will help you make delicious alternatives for regular non-vegetarian recipes like cakes, burgers, mayonnaise and many more.

The choice you have to make before getting set to read and follow this book:

Do you want to enjoy a life by eating all the junk food and meat? And then get sick and bedridden at any point of life?

Or

Do you want to eat simple-to-prepare clean vegetarian meals and live a life that does not encounter much in terms of body ailments, deficiencies, diseases, depression, etc.?

We will all die some day, but the choices we make for health reasons, are the decisions we can gift out to our future generations. Set good examples, and enjoy your first step to living a life as a Vegan and eating like you give a shit.

Chapter 1:

The truth about being Vegan

What is the truth behind being a real Vegan?

In simplest terms, being Vegan means preparing and eating purely vegetarian meals. A Vegan meal plan will not include any sort of meat, fish, poultry or game meat. It will only include food that is made or derived from plants.

That would include the leaves, shoots, roots, flowers, nuts, and fruits or various vegetables. Each country has its own variety of local vegetables that grow well and are well suited for that climate. So accordingly, many distinctive traditional vegetarian meals would have been designed in each country.

So, what does that mean to us?

Of course, it means, we have the opportunity to try cuisines from all over the world! I always recommend trying out every vegetable – and I mean fresh, not canned.

Each vegetable is unique and has a different combination of goodness piled up inside it, so you if you need a well-balanced meal, you need to take a bit of every fruit and vegetable into your daily meals.

What to keep in mind:

1. Organic products

In the supermarkets, you will be presented with a regular stock of all different vegetables of your liking. But all of these may not be necessarily good for you.

To improve the shelf life of vegetables and fruits in stores, various insecticides or pesticides would have been sprayed onto the vegetables and those fruits, before display.

Instead, go to the regular farmers market and get hold of the local organic products. They are fresh, organic, and free of chemicals, and if you are lucky, you may even get delicious products at a substantially lower price.

2. Wash Well

Now, in the event that you need to source out your daily intake of vegetables and fruits from nonorganic sellers, you just need it to wash them a bit more than the organic ones.

Just soak the fruits and vegetables for about 1 hour in a teaspoon of salt and enough water to cover them all. After one hour, drain and wash well for 3-4 times, and you will have a load of healthy vegetables at hand.

3. Fresh produce

Make sure that you enjoy fresh and crisp fruits and vegetables all the time. Do not use wilted spinach leaves, discolored root vegetables or foul smelling potatoes or cabbages or apples.

Buy just enough food items to last for a week. Not more than that, as the shelf life of organic produce is very short.

4. Variety

For those of who are still staunch meat lovers, try to borrow your favorite meat recipes and adapt those using vegetables. That way you will never get bored of eating vegetables. From this book, you will find there is no limit of humble Vegan recipes if you just think outside of the box.

Chapter 2:
What to take note of in a Well Balanced Vegan Meal Plan?

What does balanced mean to you?

I know most people will explain this as equal proportions of vitamins, proteins, minerals, fats, and carbohydrates. True that is essential, but I find just more thing equally important as the above-mentioned items.

It is none other than taste and flavors! Don't you think so?

A real healthy food may not actually taste good, and that is one of the primary concerns of people avoiding Vegan Food. So if you make it just as tasty, as it is healthy, you won't have trouble coaxing your loved ones to eat their fruits and veggies!

So, the two things that are most important in a Vegan Meal Plan are:

Goodies like minerals, vitamins, fats, etc.

And delicious food to tempt any fussy eater!

Having said that, let us take a look at what needs to be put onto a plate.

1. Calcium:

You do need to take in a lot of calcium while on a Vegan Diet. Previously, you would have supplemented it with milk and cheese and other dairy products, but now the situation is different.

Sources of Calcium:

Broccoli, Kale, figs, lady's finger, citrus fruits like oranges, collards, nuts like hazelnuts, pistachios, flax seeds and sesame seeds. You can consume a variety of dried beans like chickpeas, lentils, pinto beans, and soy beans. Almost all lentils and dried beans have calcium, so feel free to try a new variety each day. If you get a chance to purchase tempeh and tofu, those too would be important providers of calcium.

2. B12:

This is a very important vitamin that the human body needs. A very small amount is required, about 10-100mg in one day. Also, check with a doctor about your physical condition before starting any new diet or food.

Sources of B12:

B12 can be easily derived from any of the fortified kinds of foods you get in the supermarkets. For example, fortified breakfast cereals, fortified fruit juices, foods that include nutritional yeast and even tablets all are rich sources of B12 foods. You do need to consult with your doctor before consuming any such supplements.

3. Protein:

It is a fact that meat, poultry, and seafood products contain more protein in them than any vegetarian foods. Another reality is that we, human beings, do need protein to grow strong bones and stay healthy. Children and healthy elder people are in most need of protein in their diets. The former needs it because they are in their growing stage and the latter needs it to maintain their aging body.

Sources of Protein:

The most important sources of protein are hemp and the well-known soybean. They are excellent sources of protein and are also known to be starch resistant foods. That could be the reason why they are a favorite among diabetic people all around the world!

Vital sources of protein lie in lentils like dals, green grams, masoor dal, laird lentils, and many more. You can find them in the dried beans and lentils aisle in the supermarket. Remember to soak the dal in water for about 2 hours, then wash a bit and cook until they are soft when you press them with a spoon. Include tempeh and nuts into your diet apart from lentils.

4. Iron:

Iron is needed for forming blood cells in our body. If you do not have enough blood, you tend to be weak and anemic. Also, the right amount of blood is an indication of a healthy body and increases your power to fight away intruding bacteria and viruses that hover around your body all the time.

Sources of Iron:

This is one supplement that we can actually get more in vegetables compared to non-vegetarian food. It found in plenty of green leafy vegetables like spinach and many other sources are pinto beans, chickpeas, soy based products, navy beans, sesame seeds, pine nuts, cashew nuts, prunes, raisins, and sunflower seeds. Some vegetables like bok choy, turnip greens, potatoes, broccoli, and even cooked millet contain a lot of iron.

5. Fatty Acids:

By fatty acids, I mean the Omega 3 acids, which are very necessary for everyone. Omega 3 helps the blood to clot fast when you are bleeding and also prevents inflammations in the body.

Sources of Fatty Acids:

They can be found in Winter squashes, butternut squashes, pumpkins, cabbages, Brussels sprouts, arugula, Romaine leaves, and even a peculiar weed named purslane. Apart from that, you can obtain your daily dose of Omega 3 from chia seeds, flax seeds, and hemp seeds.

6. Carbohydrates:

We should remember that carbohydrates are consumed to give us energy. The body will take just the amount of carbohydrates it needs, and leave the rest to form as fat globules in our body.

Therefore, reduce your carbohydrate portions on the plate and increase the protein and healthy fats rich foods that are mentioned above.

Sources of Carbohydrates:

Carbohydrates can be found in potatoes, root vegetables, bananas, cereals, and many types of whole grains.

Chapter 3:

Exciting and Innovative Alternatives

Many Vegans complain that they cannot make certain recipes because there are no Vegan substitutes for the meat or eggs or milk mentioned in the recipes. But the fun part is, here I have mentioned a list of many ingredients that can be creatively used as clever and unsuspecting ingredients in place of non-vegetarian foods.

Egg

We do know eggs are a must in cakes, casseroles, buns, mayonnaise, and custards and many more to be mentioned.

Some of the good alternatives:

Applesauce

Ripe Bananas that are mashed well

Silken Tofu that is whizzed up in the blender or even just crumbled

Vinegar or even lemon juice: The proportion is 1 teaspoon of vinegar for 1 egg and about 1.5 teaspoons of lemon juice for 1 egg.

Nutritional Yeast added in small quantities will fluff up the dish and will bind the food well.

Meat

You can use substitutes like:

Cauliflower

Soya

Legumes

Lentils

Tempeh

Tofu

Unripe Jackfruit

Mushrooms

Potatoes

Eggplants

Unripe pumpkins

Dairy

Rice milk

Soy milk

Nut-based milk like almond or coconut milk

Cheese in the form of crumbled tofu

Soy yogurt

These are all products that you can use in meals that you are making at home. But nowadays, you can get hold of many other packaged complete Vegan products like burgers, sausages, and many other great alternatives to enjoy when you are busy or on the travel; but never make them a regular part of your cooking plans!

Chapter4:

Common Myths about Vegan Food

There are a lot of myths about Vegan food diets and that is because of the way people go about using such diets. If you do not fully understand and follow the meaning of how and what to eat for a Vegan diet, then you too are bound to hear such myths.

1. Weak bodies

This myth has popped up because Vegans generally do not eat all the different types of vegetables available on the market today. They just have their regular supply of lentils, beans, salads and soups with regular vegetables like soya, potatoes, carrots, roots and maybe some herbs. Meat, fish, and eggs contain more protein than vegetables and protein is absolutely necessary for a healthy body. If you do not include all varieties of plants and their products in your diet, you will end up with a weak body.

2. To Stay Healthy with Supplements

You must remember that all vegetables contain different combinations of vitamins, proteins, minerals, carbohydrates and only if you eat all of these, will you also become as healthy and strong. It is true that Vegans do make use of supplements and that is because of one reason.

One could be because they may not get all types of plant products in their place of residence and so they will have to compensate with the help of supplements.

3. No Cholesterol Foods

Just as much as we know cholesterol is bad for us, we need to know that is very good for us too! You must be wondering what I mean.

Well, any food for that matter is bad if taken in excess. Non-vegetarian foods contain plenty of sources of cholesterol, fats, proteins, and various minerals and still people get sick a lot. They get ill and weak because they take in too much of fats and proteins.

Vegans do need cholesterol as there are no fats in their foods. So the solution to this is eating more nuts, nut butters, and also avocados as they are rich in vegan fats.

4. Dull Meal Plans

This is a myth that was developed by people who never bothered to think of the numerous ways to make a vegetable or fruit delicious. As the world of Vegans is ever growing, it is sheer reality that ever more recipes from different cuisines around the world have been developed over the years.

Chapter 5:

Recipes- Breakfast

Okay, its day break and you are all ready to start off on another day of responsibilities, and tensions. Don't you need some edible power to get going? Check out these delectable recipes that can get you back on your legs in no time!

Buttery Vegan Buns

These buns are high power buns that are made from chickpeas and a whole lot of other vegetables.

Prep Time: 20 minutes

Cook Time: 25 minutes

Ready In: 45 minutes

Servings: 8 patties

Ingredients:

½ cup of canned chickpeas boiled and mashed

½ cup of button mushroom chopped finely

2 potatoes boiled and mashed

2 onions chopped finely

½ cup of broccoli or cauliflower riced well

1 bunch of parsley leaves finely chopped

1 teaspoon of minced garlic

Salt, thyme, pepper to taste

4 large burger buns of your choice

1 large tomato sliced thin

Hot sauce

Olive oil

Directions:

1. Combine all the ingredients in a large bowl, except the buns, tomato slices and olive oil.

2. Spray a skillet with olive oil, make patties of the mix and place on the skillet gently. Cook until golden brown on both sides.

3. Place a patty in the bun, then place a tomato slice, add hot sauce and eat warm.

Divinely Seared Honey Oat Bars

These honey bars are so delicate and will melt in your mouth. Enjoy it in the morning with a black coffee or a cup of almond milk and you can also pack it in your child's lunch box.

Prep Time: 25 minutes

Cook Time: 20 minutes

Ready In: 45 minutes

Servings: 15-20 bars

Ingredients:

2 cups of Irish oats

1.5 cups of thick coconut milk

2 cups of water

½ cup of coconut sugar

Pinch of salt

A handful of raisins and pistachios

½ cup of organic honey

½ cup of almond butter

Directions:

1. Combine the oats with coconut milk, water, and coconut sugar, salt, mix well and place in a saucepan. Cook until everything is nice and gooey.

2. Pour into a flat plate or baking tray that can fit into the freezer. Add raisins and pistachios.

3. Leave to cool in the freezer and then cut into bars.

4. Now take a skillet, add a teaspoon of butter, then place an oat bar and drizzle honey over it. Quickly flip the bar as the butter melts and ensure that the honey coats it well.

5. Take out and repeat with the rest.

Coconut and Banana infused French toast

Don't have any second thoughts about this one! Yes, it is completely Vegan and a great refreshing twist from the normal and traditional French toast.

Prep Time: 20 minutes

Cook Time: 20 minutes

Ready In: 40 minutes

Servings: 5-6 toasts

Ingredients:

4-6 slices of bread preferably old ones

1 ripe banana

½ cup of coconut milk (thick)

2 tablespoons of coconut flakes

2 tablespoons of brown sugar

Half teaspoon of nutmeg, clove, cinnamon powder each

Coconut oil

Maple syrup

Directions:

1. Put the banana and coconut milk in a blender and blend well.

2. Pour the mix into a flat bowl and add coconut flakes, brown sugar, spice powders and mix well.

3. Heat a griddle and add a teaspoon of oil on it. Dip each bread slice in the banana mix and then toast on the griddle. Flip on both sides and turn over until golden brown.

4. Serve hot with maple syrup.

Lemony Sprouted Pancakes

I have used crimson lentil sprouts and amaranth sprouts, but you can feel free to use any that you have in hand like green gram sprouts or dill sprouts.

Prep Time: 20 minutes

Cook Time: 20 minutes

Ready In: 40 minutes

Servings: 5 large pancakes or 8 small ones

Ingredients:

1.5 cups of almond milk

2 cups of whole wheat flour or any flour that you prefer

½ cup of cashew nuts soaked and ground to a fine paste

½ cup of crimson lentil sprouts

½ cup of amaranth sprouts

1 teaspoon of nutritional yeast

½ teaspoon of nutmeg powder

2 tablespoons of lemon juice

Salt to taste

4 tablespoons of organic honey

Cooking oil

Chocolate sauce or honey

Directions:

1. Mix everything in a large bowl, **except** cooking oil, and the chocolate sauce.

2. Heat a griddle, pour a bit oil and once hot, pour a ladle of the batter and cook on low heat.

3. Flip over until both sides are golden brown. Repeat until the batter is over.

4. Serve hot with chocolate sauce or just honey and some fruits.

Creamy Vegan Coconut Breakfast Bowl

A traditional recipe that uses sago pearls and the tender coconut flesh to make an extremely creamy, low fat and tasty porridge that even the fussiest of eaters will love!

Prep Time: 40 minutes

Cook Time: 20 minutes

Ready In: 60 minutes

Servings: 2 bowls

Ingredients:

¼ cup of sago pearls

½ cup of tender flesh of coconut (optional)

1.5 cups of thick coconut milk

2.5 cups of water

½ teaspoon of nutmeg powder

1 teaspoon of vanilla extract

1 large ripe cooking banana sliced thin

½ cup of coconut flakes

½ cup of cashew nuts or almond chopped

½ cup of brown sugar

2 tablespoons of vegan butter+ 3 tablespoons of cooking oil

Directions:

1. Take a large saucepan, add the 2.5 cups of water and let it boil. Once it boils, add the sago pearls and boil until it gets cooked and translucent. It will resemble tiny jelly balls.

2. Once cooked, drain the water from the cooked sago into another saucepan.

3. Place the cooked sago in a saucepan, add one cup of hot water (used to cook the sago), and the coconut milk, nutmeg powder and cook on low heat. Once it starts to boil, add the vanilla essence, stir and keep aside.

4. Now in a frying pan, add the butter and oil, then add the bananas slices and fry until golden and just crispy on the outside. Add the coconut flakes, chopped cashew nuts, brown sugar and stir until sugar has melted and everything is coated well with the sugary syrup. Add a pinch of salt, mix and pour this mix into the porridge. You can add the tender coconut at this point and serve warm or cold. Tender coconut flesh needs no cooking.

Chapter 6:
Recipes- Lunch

It is noon time and you must be feeling tired and hungry. Why not think about rolling your sleeves and making these heavenly lip smackers in a jiffy?

Peppery Bulgur Wraps

For these bulgur wraps, red peppers have been used not only for the pepper flavor but for the vibrant color too. The wraps are made our of whole wheat wraps, but if you like rice wrappers they too will taste very nice.

Prep Time: 40 minutes

Cook Time: 15 minutes

Ready In: 55 minutes

Servings: 4-6 wraps

Ingredients:

6 large red peppers chopped

2 garlic cloves

½ teaspoon of paprika

Salt to taste

½ cup of olive oil

3 soya meatless sausages cut into thin slices

½ cup of bulgur

½ cup of pinto beans

3 garlic cloves chopped finely chopped

½ teaspoon chili flakes

4 shallots chopped

½ cup of chopped parsley

6 wheat tortillas

Directions:

1. Take a large saucepan, add the pinto beans and 3 garlic cloves and sufficient to cover and cook at a low flame until they are soft and well cooked. Now pour about ½ cup of warm water, add bulgur, chili flakes and salt to taste and switch off the gas. Wait for the bulgur to absorb all the water and let it bloom and become soft. Then open and fluff up with a fork.

2. Now take a saucepan and add the red peppers, 2 garlic cloves, paprika and salt and boil until the peppers are soft. Leave to cool a bit and then blend in the blender with the ½ cup of olive oil.

3. Now heat the tortillas, and begin preparing the wraps. Meanwhile lightly fry the meatless sausages and keep aside.

4. Spread a large tablespoon of the pepper paste, and then add the bulgur and bean mix, sausages, shallots, and some parsley and wrap carefully.

5. Your wraps are ready to be munched away.

Sweet and sour Tempeh with Garlic Brown Rice

Tempeh is a very source of protein for Vegans. They are easy to make and blends with almost all spices and you can fry, bake, or boil them as you like.

Prep Time: 40 minutes

Cook Time: 15 minutes

Ready In: 55 minutes

Servings: 4 persons

Ingredients:

7 ounces of tempeh cut into 1 inch cubes

1.5 cups of brown rice cooked

4 garlic cloves

1 large onion chopped finely

4 tablespoons of sesame oil

2 teaspoons of soy sauce

2 teaspoons of honey

1 teaspoon of vinegar or lime juice

2 teaspoons of tomato ketchup

¼ cup of broccoli flowerets

¼ cup of chopped mushrooms

¼ cup of baby corn

2 cups of chopped kale

¼ cup of peanuts

Directions:

1. Take a bowl, add tempeh with the soy sauce, honey, vinegar, and mix and marinate for 10 minutes.

2. In a frying pan, add sesame oil, and once hot, fry the tempeh slightly until golden brown on all sides. Keep aside.

3. In the hot oil, add garlic, onions, stir on high heat. Quickly, add the mushrooms and stir fry for about 5 minutes until cooked.

4. Then add the baby corn, kale, peanuts, and finally the broccoli and toss well in the hot oil. You can add more oil, if it gets too dry.

5. Now add tempeh and the brown rice mix well and finally add salt and ketchup and toss and serve hot. It will equally be good when it is cold or hot.

Yam with Ginger Coconut Curry

Yam is a rich source of minerals and vitamins and it is especially good for women. This dish is great to be served with a pile of hot white rice and some fresh greens.

Prep Time: 12 minutes

Cook Time: 20 minutes

Ready In: 32 minutes

Servings: 4 persons

Ingredients:

1 cup of yam skinned and cubed

1 cup of cauliflower flowerets

1 teaspoon of chili powder

½ teaspoon of turmeric powder

½ teaspoon of garam masala

Salt to taste

2 teaspoons of minced ginger

1 large onion finely chopped

2 green chilies slit into half

¼ teaspoon of mustard seeds

¼ teaspoon of cumin seeds

2 cups of thin coconut milk

1 bunch of chopped coriander leaves

2 tablespoons of cooking oil

Directions:

1. Take a bowl, add the yam with the chili powder, turmeric power, garam masala, and salt and mix well. Place in a saucepan with about ½ cup of water and boil on a low flame, until soft. Keep covered to cook fast.

2. In a large saucepan, add cooking oil, then the mustard seeds and cumin seeds. Once the seeds start to crackle, stay away from it for 4-5 seconds. Then add the onions, ginger, and green chilies and stir on low heat. Now add the cauliflower and stir and leave to cook on a low flame.

3. Once cauliflower is cooked, add the boiled yam, and coconut milk, salt to taste and stir well. Let it boil and finally add the coriander leaves. The dish is ready.

4. Serve with some steaming hot rice or some fresh whole wheat bread.

Curried Spinach and Tofu Pita Pockets

Have you ever tried scrambled tofu? Well, it tastes just like scrambled eggs and of course way healthier than eggs!

Prep Time: 12 minutes

Cook Time: 20 minutes

Ready In: 32 minutes

Servings: 4 persons

Ingredients:

2 cups of fresh spinach

8 ounces of crumbled silken tofu

1 teaspoon of curry powder

1 medium onion chopped finely

1 tomato chopped roughly

2 tablespoons of cooking oil

Salt to taste

2 large pita breads cut into half to make pockets

Directions:

1. Take a skillet, add oil, then add the onions, tomato and stir on high heat, then add the tofu, curry powder and spinach, salt and stir on medium heat. Stir till everything is well combined.

2. Scoop the tofu mix and fill into the pita pockets and your lunch is ready!

Soy Chili glazed Tofu over Noodles

Rice noodles have been used here and they have been drenched in a rich sauce made from tofu and a lot of other vegetables.

Prep Time: 12 minutes

Cook Time: 20 minutes

Ready In: 32 minutes

Servings: 4 persons

Ingredients:

2 cups of tofu cubed in 1 inch cubes

8 ounces of rice noodles boiled and kept to cool

1 teaspoon of chili flakes

2 tablespoons of soy sauce

2 teaspoons of maple syrup

1 teaspoon of cayenne pepper

2 tablespoons of lime juice

2 tablespoons of miso paste

2 cups of vegetable broth

½ cup of toasted peanuts lightly chopped

5 tablespoons of sesame oil

½ cup of cooked chopped mushrooms

½ cup of boiled peas

½ cup of shredded cabbage

½ cup of bean sprouts

½ cup of green pepper chopped finely

½ cup of chopped cilantro

Directions:

1. Take a frying pan, and lightly fry the tofu cubes until slightly brown on all sides.

2. Take a saucepan; add the vegetable broth, chili flakes, soy sauce, cayenne pepper, maple syrup, and boil at low heat. Once it has boiled, take about ½ cup of the boiling liquid in a cup, and dissolve the miso paste. Pour it back into the saucepan and finally pour the lime juice. Leave to cool a bit.

3. Once the sauce has cooled a bit, add the peanuts, sesame oil, mushrooms, peas, cabbage, bean sprouts, green pepper, salt to taste and finally add the noodles and cilantro and toss well.

4. Serve hot or cold.

Chapter 7:

Recipes- Cravings

Two main meals are over and are you in the mood for some spicy or sweet Vegan bites. Try these simple recipes, which can be prepared and eaten for picnics, kiddy parties, movie time and even family meetings.

Millet Onion Crunch

These are wonderful crunchy cravings, which can be stocked up in containers and will remain fresh for 3-4 days.

Prep Time: 12 minutes

Cook Time: 20 minutes

Ready In: 32 minutes

Servings: 25- 30 persons

Ingredients:

1 cup of good quality millet

3 cups of water

2 large onions finely chopped

1 small red pepper finely chopped

4- 5 tablespoons of rice flour

¼ teaspoon of garlic powder

Salt to taste

Cooking oil

Directions:

1. Cook the millet with 3 cups of water and salt until soft. Leave to cool.

2. Now mix the cooked millet, onions, red peppers, rice flour, and garlic powder, salt to taste and mix well.

3. Apply cooking oil on a baking tray and then press the millet mix into the baking tray. Spray with cooking oil on top of the millet mix.

4. Bake for 20 minutes at 300F until the top is golden brown.

Coconut Cherry Crispys

These crispys do not require any cooking and can stay crispy for about 3 days. If you store in the refrigerator, it will do well for about 10 days.

Prep Time: 15 minutes

Cook Time: -

Ready In: 15 minutes

Servings: 25- 30 balls

Ingredients:

2 cups of Rice Crispys

¾ cup of almond butter

¼ cup of coconut flakes

¼ cup of pitted and halved cherries

¼ cup of cocoa nibs

¼ cup of honey

½ teaspoon of mint extract

Directions:

1. Place all the ingredients in a large bowl and mix well. Then butter your hands with some oil or almond butter, and roll out the mix into small balls.

2. Place the balls in the freezer section for one hour and then you can serve chewy balls at once.

No Bake Cinnamon Flax Bars

When you can get no bake snacks to fix those hunger pangs, wouldn't it be great? Of course, lesser work and lesser use of energy!

Prep Time: 10 minutes

Cook Time: 10 minutes

Ready In: 20 minutes

Servings: 20-25 bars

Ingredients:

1 cup of flax seed powder

¾ cup of sunflower seed butter

¼ cup of wheat germ

¼ cup of raisins

1 teaspoon of cinnamon powder

¾ cup of protein powder of your choice

5 tablespoons of brown rice syrup

Chocolate sauce (optional)

Directions:

1. Place everything in a large bowl, except the chocolate sauce.

2. Mix well and spread evenly and firmly on a baking tray.

3. Place in the fridge for 30 minutes, then drizzle chocolate sauce over it and then again keep for 30 minutes in the fridge.

4. Take out, cut into bars and serve.

Blueberry and Cashew Pudding

A complete health pudding that can be made overnight and you can scoop up a cold bowl of this yummy pudding when you feel hungry.

Prep Time: 10 minutes

Cook Time: 10 minutes

Ready In: 20 minutes

Servings: 4-7 persons

Ingredients:

1 cup of cooked oats

½ cup of cashews soaked for 30 minutes and pureed to a paste

1 cup of fresh blueberries

2 cups of almond milk

1 teaspoon of vanilla extract

½ cup of maple syrup

Directions:

1. Place everything in a large saucepan, and boil at a low heat.

2. Once the blueberries have become soft, take off from gas and leave to cool.

3. Enjoy cold.

Mint Cheez

A great variety to surprise folks at home or for any party! Try them and you will love the new flavors that are combined in them.

Prep Time: 10 minutes

Cook Time: 10 minutes

Ready In: 20 minutes

Servings: 12-15 balls

Ingredients:

1 cup of silken tofu

1 cup of chopped mint leaves

1 teaspoon of paprika

Salt to taste

½ cup rice flour+ water

Oil for frying

Directions:

1. Place tofu, mint leaves, salt and paprika in a bowl and mix well and form small balls.

2. Make a thick with the rice flour and water.

3. Heat oil in a saucepan. Once hot, dip each ball in the rice batter and fry in the hot oil.

4. Serve with tomato ketchup or some hot sauce.

Chapter 8:
Recipes- Vegan Protein Shakes

Protein Shakes should be a must in every diet plan, as there will be days when you are not in the mood to do some extensive cooking or perhaps don't have the time or don't feel quite right. So, if you have a few tummy filling recipes, it will keep going through the day.

Robust Kale with Banana Protein Shake

Kale will give all the iron and calcium and bananas will lend in tons of potassium, and this is what everyone needs in the morning before a workout.

Prep Time: 10 minutes

Cook Time: 10 minutes

Ready In: 20 minutes

Servings: 2 large glasses

Ingredients:

1 cup of kale leaves, no stalks

1 ripe banana

1 cup almond milk

2 tablespoons honey

1 cup cold water

1 teaspoon of vanilla extract

2 scoops of vanilla DailyBurn Fuel-6

Directions:

1. Place everything in a blender and blend well.

2. Pour into tall glasses and enjoy.

Strawberries with Hemp Protein Shake

Strawberries along with hemp will not give a vibrant color, but will supply all the antioxidants, proteins and vitamins needed for a person, especially for Vegan person.

Prep Time: 10 minutes

Cook Time: 10 minutes

Ready In: 20 minutes

Servings: 2 large glasses

Ingredients:

1 cup of hulled strawberries

2 tablespoons of hemp powder

3 tablespoons of palm sugar

1 cup of any nut milk you like

1 cup of cold water

½ cup of rolled cooked oats

Directions:

1. Place everything in a blender and blend well.

2. Pour into tall glasses and enjoy.

Blueberries with Prunes Protein Shake

Kick start the bright mornings with some protein boosting drinks and it is bound to make you energetic and happy all day.

Prep Time: 10 minutes

Cook Time: 10 minutes

Ready In: 20 minutes

Servings: 2 large glasses

Ingredients:

1 cup of cleaned blueberries

½ cup of prunes soaked in water- 6 hours

½ cup of cashews soaked in water- 6 hours

4 tablespoons of chia seeds

2 cups of thin coconut milk

2 scoops of protein powder you prefer

Directions:

1. Place everything in a blender and blend well.

2. Pour into tall glasses and enjoy.

Apples with Banana Spinach Protein Shake

You deserve a fruity delight to take the hidden challenges of the day ahead. Don't you think so?

Prep Time: 10 minutes

Cook Time: 10 minutes

Ready In: 20 minutes

Servings: 2 large glasses

Ingredients:

2 apples skinned and chopped

1 ripe banana

1 cup of baby spinach

½ cup of barley

4 tablespoons of coconut sugar

2.5 cups of water

2 scoops of vanilla protein powder

Directions:

1. Soak the barley in water for about 10 hours, drain it, and boil with 2 cups of water until very soft. Blend well and strain. You get your barley milk.

2. Place barley milk, apples, banana, spinach, coconut sugar, protein powder, and water in a blender and blend well.

3. Pour into tall glasses and enjoy.

Kiwi with Pomegranate Dates Protein Shake

There is always time to make some so exotic as these proteins drink that includes some kiwi and pomegranate.

Prep Time: 10 minutes

Cook Time: 10 minutes

Ready In: 20 minutes

Servings: 2 large glasses

Ingredients:

2 small kiwis skinned and chopped

1 ripe banana

1 cup of pomegranate seeds

1 tablespoon of flax seeds

1 tablespoon of hemp powder

¼ cup of mint leaves

4 dates pitted and soaked in water

2. 5 cups of soy milk or water

Directions:

1. Place everything in a blender and blend well.

2. Pour into tall glasses and enjoy.

Chapter 9:

Recipes- Dinner

The day has finally come to an end and finally you made it through the day! There are quite simple recipes that can feed a crowd in here.

Killer Vegan Sloppy Pasta

Vegan Pasta made in sloppy Joes style is a real hit

Prep Time: 15 minutes

Cook Time: 20 minutes

Ready In: 35 minutes

Servings: 4-6 people

Ingredients:

8 ounces of vegan pasta

1 cup of chopped zucchini

1 cup of chopped mushroom

½ cup of chopped tempeh

½ cup of red peppers and green peppers each

½ cup of chopped carrot and peas each

1 cup of tomato puree

1 cup of chopped onions

2 teaspoons of garlic paste

1 tablespoon of hot sauce and soy sauce each

1 teaspoon of rosemary, pepper and thyme each

5 tablespoons of cooking oil

Salt to taste

Directions:

1. Place a large skillet on the heat and pour oil. Once hot, add garlic, onions, tomato puree and stir until the onions sweats.

2. Then add everything else except the pasta and stir quickly on high heat. Cover for 10 minutes until everything is cooked.

3. Adjust seasonings and add pasta and stir and serve hot.

Mushroom Celery Curry

An exotic curry that uses simple vegetables to lend a truly nostalgic flavor. Enjoy with rice.

Prep Time: 15 minutes

Cook Time: 30 minutes

Ready In: 45 minutes

Servings: 4-6 people

Ingredients:

5 tablespoons of cooking oil

Salt to taste

3 stalks of celery

½ cup of scallions chopped

1 inch of ginger peeled and minced

2 large potatoes skin removed, chopped

1 cup of chopped mushrooms

1 cup of cauliflower flowerets

1 cup of chopped unripe jackfruit flesh

2 cups of thick coconut milk+ 1 cup of water

½ teaspoon of nutmeg, pepper, cinnamon powder each

Directions:

1. Heat a large saucepan, add oil and then add all the ingredients in it, mix and close the lid. Cook at a low heat for 30 minutes.

2. Serve hot with rice and salad.

Roasted Eggplants with Cauliflower drenched Pasta

All basic ingredients and there is nothing that could go wrong here!

Prep Time: 15 minutes

Cook Time: 30 minutes

Ready In: 45 minutes

Servings: 4-6 people

Ingredients:

2 large eggplants

1 small cauliflower

1 cup of silken tofu

2 cups of coconut milk

8 ounces of boiled Vegan pasta

4-5 torn basil leaves

Cooking oil

Sea salt, chili flakes

2 teaspoons of lime juice

Directions:

1. Place about 2 cups of water in a saucepan, add salt, and let it boil.

2. Meanwhile, clean the cauliflower and break into small pieces. Add into boiling water for 8 minutes, boil, and then strain and keep aside.

3. Roast the eggplants with sea salt and chili flakes at 300F for about 15 minutes.

4. Blend the cauliflower with silken tofu and coconut milk until smooth.

5. Take a deep baking pan, add the pasta, roasted eggplants, and cauliflower sauce, add seasonings and bake for 20 minutes at 250F until the top has become golden brown. Serve with basil leaves.

Vegan Wild Garlic Stir Fry

Stir fries are crisp and fresh and great for any time of the day.

Prep Time: 15 minutes

Cook Time: 30 minutes

Ready In: 45 minutes

Servings: 4 people

Ingredients:

2 cups of boiled wild rice

½ cup of broccoli flowerets

½ cup of baby corn

½ cup of snow peas

½ cup of carrots

½ cup of red and green peppers each

½ cup of peanuts

2 tablespoons of soy sauce

1 teaspoon of vinegar

1 teaspoon of brown sugar

2 tablespoon of green chili sauce

¼ cup of sesame oil

1 cup of chopped shallots

5 garlic cloves minced

Directions:

1. Take a large wok, or frying pans, add oil. Once hot, add garlic and onions and stir quickly on high heat.

2. Then add the vegetables one by one, then the sauces and finally the cooked rice.

3. Stir well on high heat and serve hot.

Quinoa Miso Celery Soup

A filing and feel good soup for any time of the year. You can use fennel instead of celery of you like.

Prep Time: 15 minutes

Cook Time: 30 minutes

Ready In: 45 minutes

Servings: 4-6 people

Ingredients:

10 cups of water

1 cup of uncooked good quality quinoa

5 stalks of celery chopped

5 garlic cloves chopped

2 large onions chopped

6 large tomatoes pureed

2 tablespoons of miso paste

½ cup of cooked pinto beans and pureed

Salt and pepper to taste

Directions:

1. Take a large pot, add 1 tablespoon of cooking oil, then add garlic, onions, and tomatoes and stir well for 5 minutes on high heat.

2. Add broth or water and let it boil. Now, add celery, pinto bean paste and boil for 10 minutes. Add salt. Now, take about 5 tablespoons of the soup in a bowl and mix the miso paste in it. Pour back the entire mix in the soup.

3. Add quinoa and switch off the gas and wait for it to absorb the flavors and get cooked.

4. Serve hot.

Chapter 10:

Recipes- Desserts

A good meal has to end with a dessert. Vegan meals have wonderful options for simple desserts, so why not enjoy low cal sweet surprises after an energizing multivitamin meal?

Peanut Balls

Simple and not too sweet for the tooth

Prep Time: 30 minutes

Cook Time: 10 minutes

Ready In: 40 minutes

Servings: 10 people

Ingredients:

2 cups of powdered peanuts

½ cup of coconut oil

¾ cup of brown sugar

Salt

Directions:

1. Take a large saucepan, add oil, peanut powder, and a pinch of salt and mix well. Heat it slowly and keep stirring. Once the peanut aroma comes, add the brown sugar and combine well. Take off from gas.

2. Leave to cool for 10 minutes. Then apply oil on your hands, take big spoonfuls of the mix and roll in your hands. You can roll as long as it not too hot to touch. But it should still be warm. If it doesn't come together, add a little bit coconut or almond milk.

3. Store in the refrigerator.

Raspberry Ice- cream

Use any fruit you like, it will taste refreshing and nutritious too!

Prep Time: 10 minutes

Cook Time: -

Ready In: 6 hours (freezing) 10 minutes

Servings: 4 people

Ingredients:

2 cups of raspberries

½ cup of vanilla protein powder

¾ cup of coconut sugar

2 cups of thick coconut milk

Directions:

1. Blend everything in a blender and pour in a freezer compact container.

2. Leave to freeze and then scoop when it is time to serve.

Coconut Mint Jello

Great for all mint lovers

Prep Time: 10 minutes + 4 hours

Cook Time: 10 minutes

Ready In: 20 minutes+ 4 hours

Servings: 4 people

Ingredients:

2.5 cups of almond milk

2 tablespoons of Vegan gelatin

2 tablespoons of peppermint powder

5 tablespoons of honey

Directions:

1. Heat the almond milk in a saucepan and add the gelatin, stir until melted.

2. Cool the milk and place in a airtight container, along with the peppermint powder, and honey, mix well and leave to set in the fridge for about 4 hours.

3. Serve cold after a meal

Papaya Delight

A cooling combo of papaya and strawberries with choco chips

Prep Time: 10 minutes + 4 hours

Cook Time: 10 minutes

Ready In: 20 minutes+ 4 hours

Servings: 4 people

Ingredients:

1 cup of cashew milk

2 cups of Red Papaya cubes

2 cups of strawberries hulled and cut into small chunks

2 tablespoons of cacao nibs

5 tablespoons of maple syrup

Directions:

1. Blend papaya and cashew milk well.

2. Add strawberries, cacao nibs and honey and mix well.

3. Keep in freezer for 4 hours, until ready to serve.

Blueberry Vegan Cheesecake

A healthy version of a cheesecake and absolutely no dairy in it!

Prep Time: 10 minutes + 4 hours

Cook Time: 10 minutes

Ready In: 20 minutes+ 4 hours

Servings: 4 people

Ingredients:

1 cup of thick coconut milk

1 cup of thick cashew paste (Soak 35-40 cashew nuts in water for 1 hour and then grind)

1.5 cups of blueberries

5 tablespoons of coconut sugar+ pinch of salt

½ cup of maple syrup

¼ teaspoon of nutmeg powder, cinnamon powder each

½ cup of wheat germ

½ cup of flax seeds

½ cup of oat powder

½ cup of fortified corn flakes powdered

¾ cup of nut butter or coconut oil

Directions:

1. Mix wheat germ, flax seeds, oat powder, corn flakes powder, and nut butter and mix well. Press this mix firmly into a deep wide pan and keep in fridge.

2. Beat the cashew paste, coconut milk, nutmeg and cinnamon powder and maple syrup well with a spatula. Then pour onto the wheat germ crust base and keep in the fridge to set for one hour.

3. Next, place the blueberries in a saucepan and cook at low heat. Once it starts to warm, smash the berries a bit and add coconut sugar and pinch of salt. Take off from gas and let it cool completely.

4. Pour the berry mix onto the cashew mix and let it set for 3 hours in the fridge.

5. Cut into wedges and serve.

Conclusion

The Vegan Meal plan is in reality a very simple one to follow. It is true that in the beginning you may find it hard to substitute meat dishes for 100% vegan dishes, but when you think about the pros and cons of both, you will find it easier to make your decision.

My personal advice to you: Always start by making small batches when you try new recipes or combinations. If you like it, then you can go ahead and make a large batch.

There are no hard and fast rules in cooking, but stick by these two rules. Make sure you are having a balanced meal. A bit of everything from carbohydrates to vitamins, proteins, fats, and minerals should be on your plate.

And second, ensure that the food is tasty, not just healthy. If it is not tasty, the mind and taste buds will reject it and then there is no use taking so much care in preparing them. So make sure whatever you cook is irresistible to your palate!

I hope you enjoyed the book just as much as I enjoyed giving this precious knowledge to you. Enjoy good quality Vegan food, live life, and eat like you give a shit!

www.ingramcontent.com/pod-product-compliance
Lightning Source LLC
Chambersburg PA
CBHW050755290526
45792CB00008B/2196